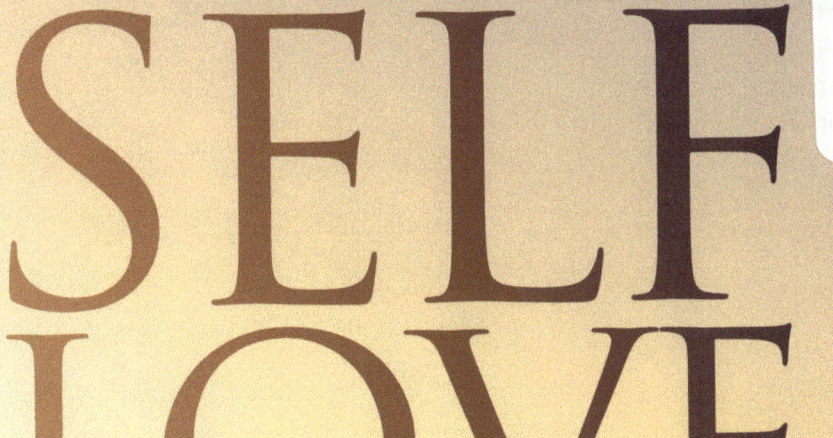

SELF LOVE

Heart Based Education™
Module One

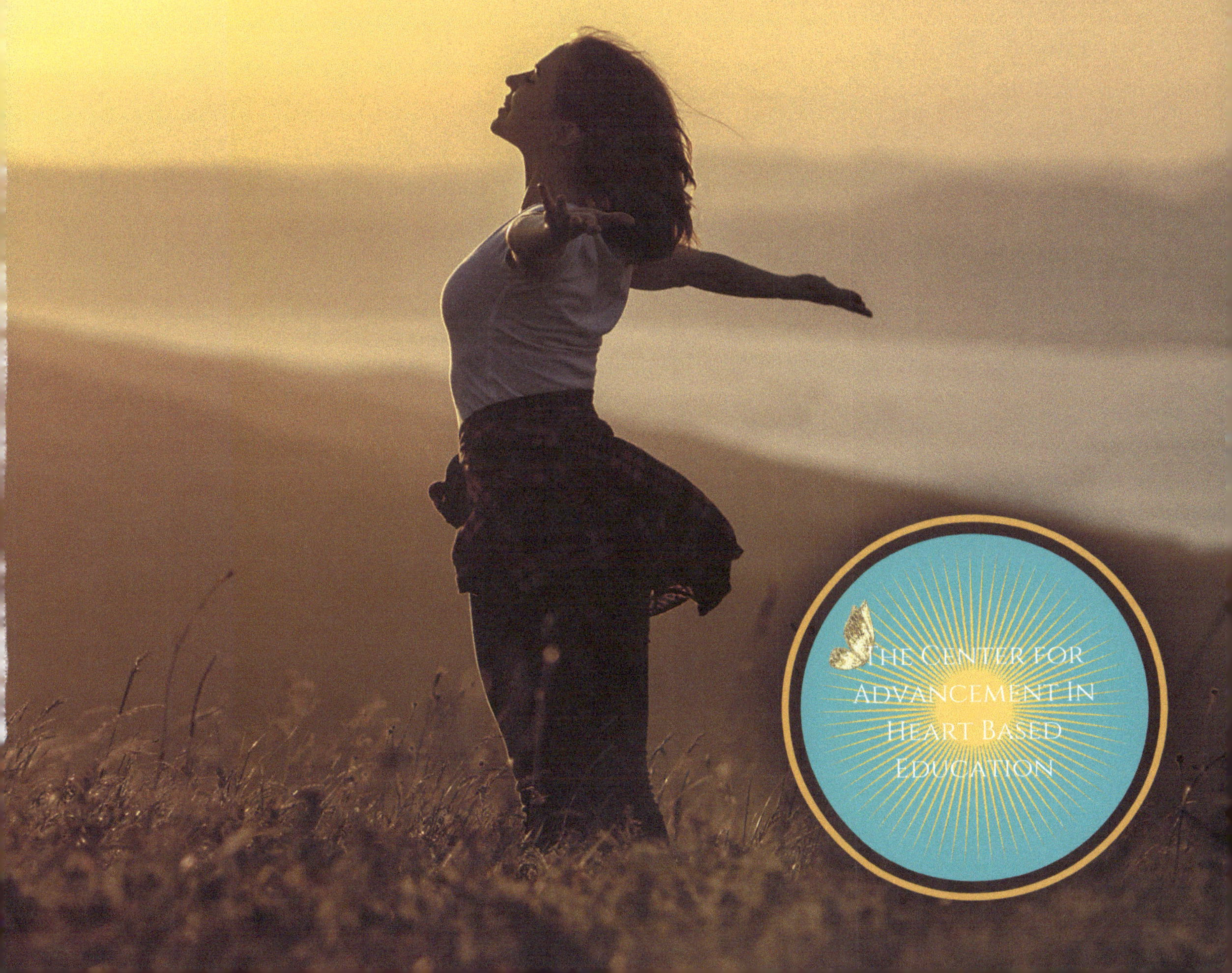

THE CENTER FOR
ADVANCEMENT IN
HEART BASED
EDUCATION

Primix Publishing
East Brunswick Office Evolution
1 Tower Center Boulevard, Ste 1510
East Brunswick, NJ 08816
www.primixpublishing.com
Phone: 1-800-538-5788

Published by Primix Publishing: 10/10/2025

ISBN: 979-8-89194-554-8(sc)
ISBN: 979-8-89194-555-5(e)

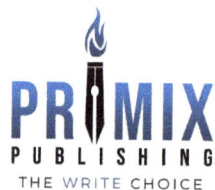

PRIMIX
PUBLISHING
THE WRITE CHOICE

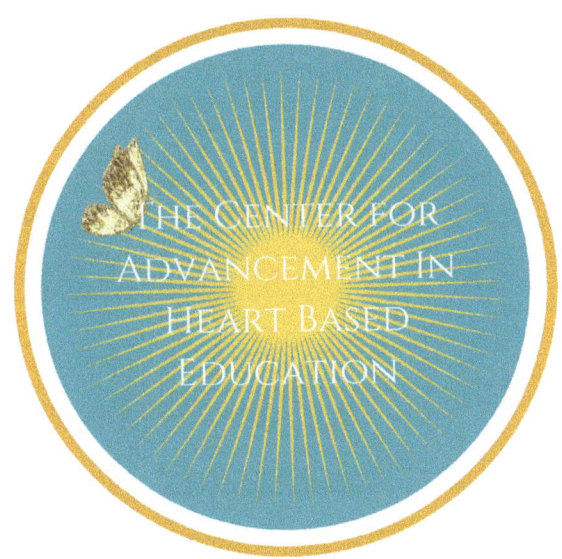

Self-Love, Module One: Here we lay the foundation for empowering individuals—educators and learners alike—to cultivate self-love as a core component of their personal, professional and educational growth. This module centers on the anchor to the heart, a practice of connecting deeply with one's heart space, the source of inner peace, wisdom, and authentic guidance.

Through guided activations, participants are led to connect with their hearts, through an experiential journey where they learn to access their heart connection. This begins the process and trust of their inner guidance system, developing a sense of self-awareness, acceptance, and connection to their innate worth. The module and workshop provides tools and strategies for fostering self-love, emphasizing the transformative power of heart-based practices in shaping emotional resilience, empathy, and social harmony.

Participants experience:

1. The Seed of Light/Heart Connection: A meditation/activation,an autonomous and sovereign freedom practice to connect to the heart's wisdom and align with unconditional self love.

2. Inner Guidance Cultivation: A series of guided written and creative reflections and discoveries to tap into personal self trust, understanding and self-compassion.

3. Practical Integration: Extension practices and tools that carry far beyond the actual workshop/module. Tools and approaches for educators, participants and learners to experience, embody, model and nurture self-love in themselves and their lives.

This module and workshop are the foundational part of a stacking experience and growth process, empowering participants to integrate these heart-based practices into their professional and personal lives, creating ripples of positivity in self, family, community and the world.

More about The Center for Advancement in Heart Based Education and our modules:

Our **eight stacking training modules** are designed to stand alone as a workshop, or class, and are a part of a certification opportunity with The Center for Advancement in Heart Based Education. The modules were created to seamlessly partner with any learning environment, offering tools to cultivate personal growth, emotional balance, and interpersonal connection. These modules create a framework of tools and techniques for personal and professional development, to build healthier relationships with self, and our communities while addressing each person's gifts, mission and purpose, with support on the day to day for navigating the challenges of life, while supporting optimum mental health, resolving attention issues, and upholding the delivery of trauma informed recovery, and whole person education.

Through interactive workshops, embodiment techniques, and transformative activations, we guide participants to connect with their hearts, discover their inner gifts, and align with their life purpose. Together, we aim to create a future of compassionate, thriving individuals and communities. Next visit Be The Medicine; The Medicine Wheel Exploration Technique, Module Two.

Find out more here: www.HeartBasedED.org

SELF LOVE WHEEL THE CENTER FOR ADVANCEMENT IN HEART BASED EDUCATION™

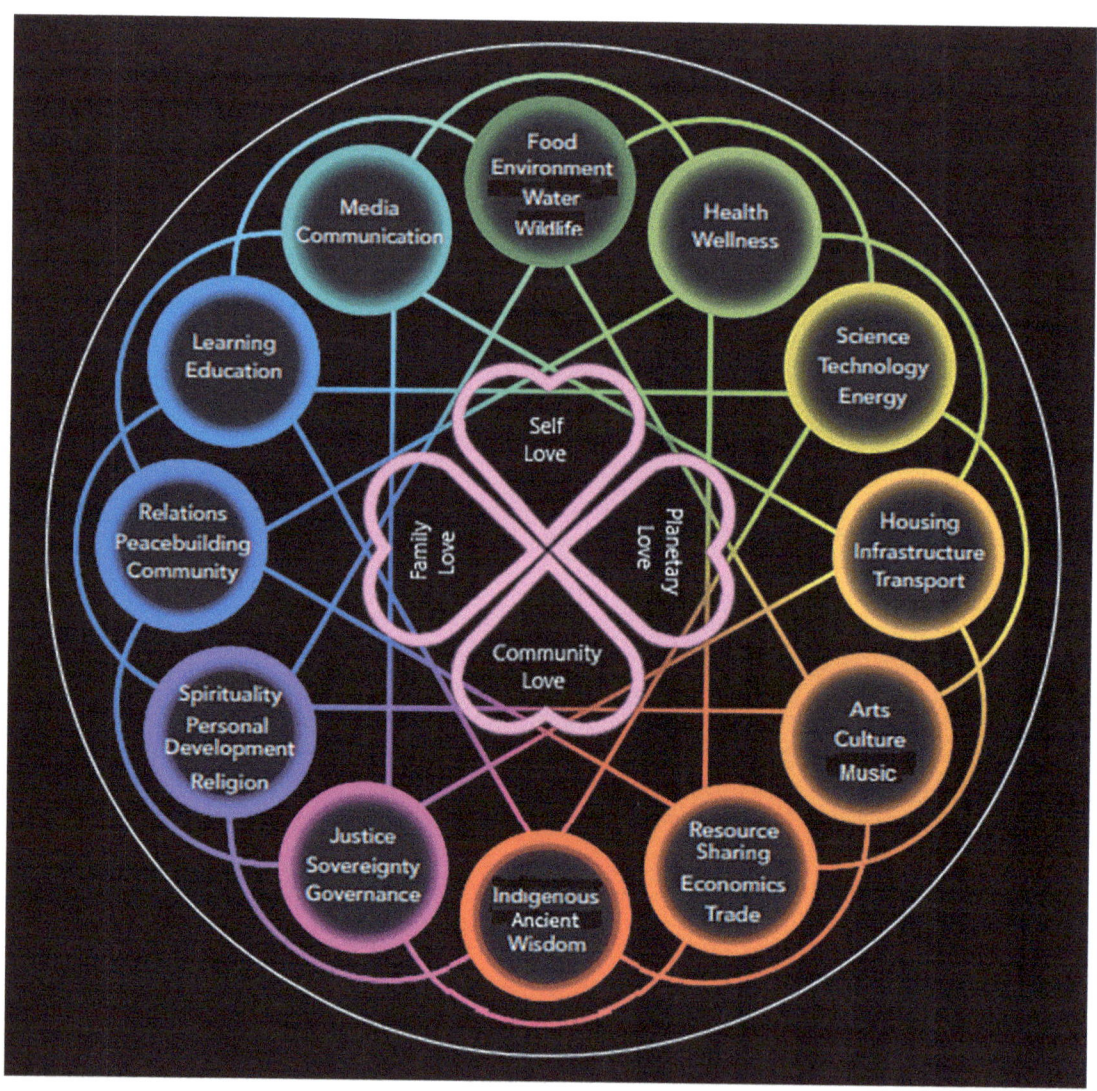

SELF LOVE

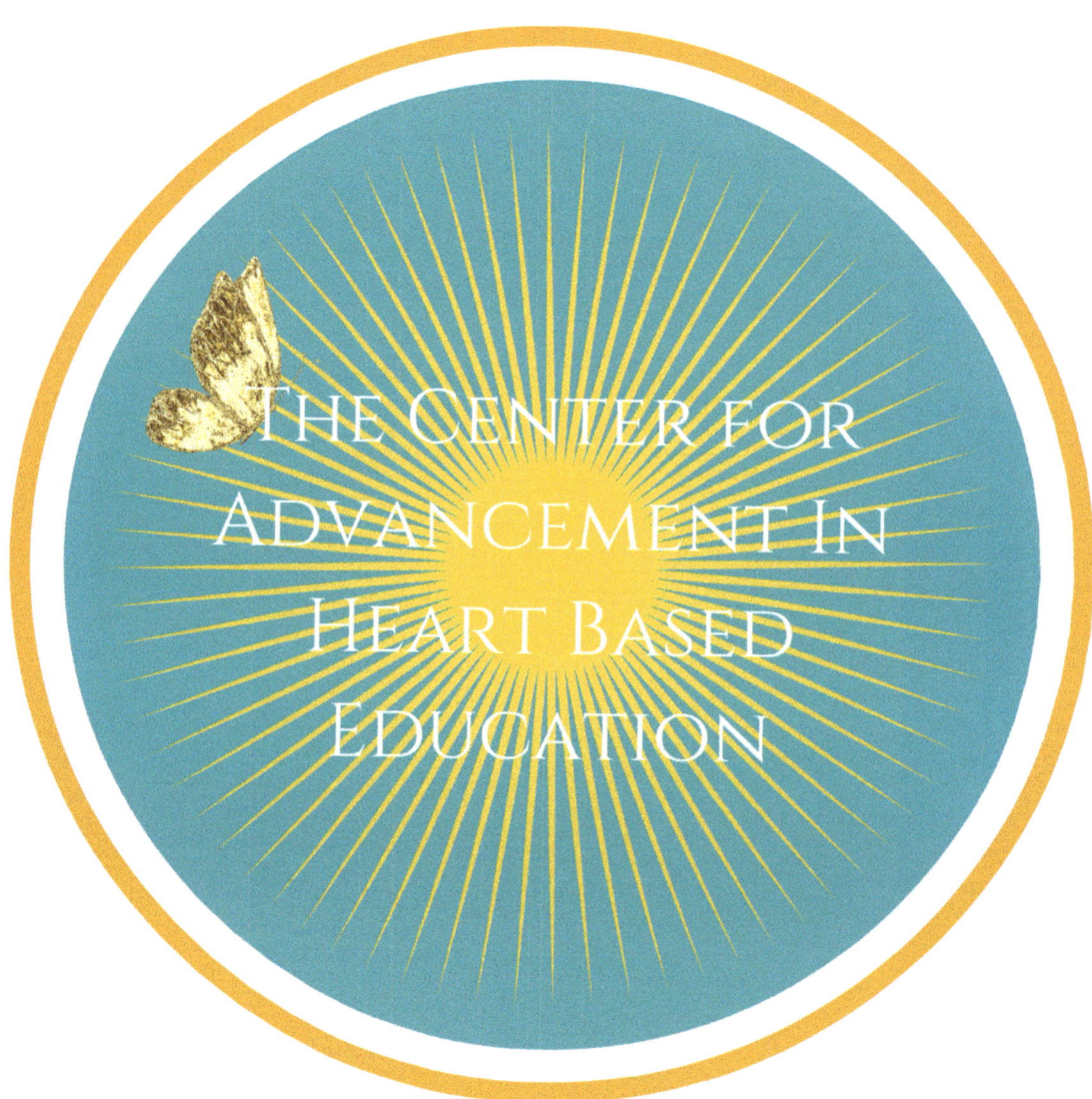

The Center for Advancement In Heart Based Education

Heart Based Education
2nd Edition

MODULE ONE

Forward:

Self love is something that we cultivate within ourselves. The landscape of society and education are transforming along with us. We realize the importance of Heart Based Education™. Through understanding self in relation to, family, community and the world, focused on our own personal self love development, we begin to create a different landscape that works for us individually, and because of that, works for others. The following manual is a turnkey guide to and through embodiment practices, tools and techniques that have been tested and proven effective over the past 30 years in a variety of education settings internationally, reaching all ages and beliefs.

We have spent many years training bodies and minds. It is time to focus on the heart.

The Center for Advancement in Heart Based Education™ Mission:
We are international educators and learners implementing Heart Based Practices, Tools and Techniques, we raise the bar of/for love, care and respect for ourselves and all our relations.

Curriculum Series Heart Based Education: The Center for Advancement in Heart Based Education™.

All Rights Reserved 2017 ISBN: 9798307942994 Published by The Center for Advancement in Social Emotional™ Learning/Heart Based Education 2025

Resource Materials and Certifications at www.HeartBasedED.org

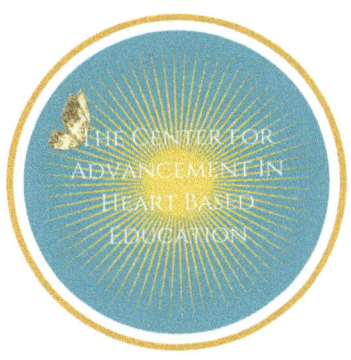

Self Love Turn Key Guide: Module One™

Welcome

This is one of the most important things you have ever done for yourself and for another person. Here we get to know ourselves, come to understand how to love ourselves, and how to facilitate that with anyone with whom we have the opportunity to share in the future. We are going to learn about **safe and brave space and self love practices**, for ourselves and as a community of humans. The Center for Advancement has set some preliminary guidelines to help you understand the process,and to support you in creating your own set of guidelines that works for you and those in your space. We set guidelines so safe and brave space can be felt for all to express themselves and their truth. As active participants in our lives, and as potential facilitators, and educators, it is our job to **"Hold Space"**, for ourselves, for our loved ones, for our communities, and for our world. As we face this new world reality, we need new ways to connect and feel safe to explore self and our relations with family, community and the world.

Activity #1: "**Holding Space**: To "hold space' is the first teaching. It is an energy we embody when we decide we will include others in an activity in our space. In that space imagine and hold intention, that the space is safe, we imagine and hold intention for the best for all involved. We are active and supportive listeners, engaging in the activity and with the participants at all times. We become the embodiment of our values, of our love, from our care and from our respect for ourselves and others. Empowered presence.Then we work as the platform, a literal island or stage, from which safe space emanates. It becomes a safe place that extends out from us, and all around us, and it is felt by all involved.

As we begin to explore, understand,and finally teach about self love, we must include each person within our group as a unique and important part of the process. We begin this by calling in each person to form a circle and,now that we are internationally on-line, a virtual circle or an expanded circle of community can be formed.

After everyone is assembled, we call on each individual to activate in love, care, and respect, of supportive and active listening. We explain that to be supportive and active listeners, there are guidelines of the circle/process. Here are the guidelines for a safe and brave space circle:

1) We do not speak out of turn
2) Each person's time to share is theirs to share, and we respect others' time who are listening, as we are respected while we share
3) No feedback is necessary
4) We are all here showing up in the moment

Within this we then guide and inform in order to share our truth.

What is it to love ourselves, to care for self, to respect self?"

This is our theme for this module. And what we will be exploring.

Principles to holding a safe and brave space circle:

When we hold a circle - one where each individual feels loved, cared for, and respected, and part of a greater whole - we set a tone for a new way of living. We model. "This is a no judgment zone." Each person has their own sacred space to speak. As light facilitators we make sure of this, always responding positively, and thanking the person for sharing with us.

Acknowledgement is key. At the end of the circle (after everyone has shared), we have a moment of gratitude for our safe and brave space, and we share our gratitude openly and give thanks that each person participated in this safe and brave space. Then we share with our participants that we move out into the day from this safe and brave space. We acknowledge it is a gift to take what was created and learned with us out into the world.

Beginning a safe and brave space circle:

One word to describe how you are feeling today? (This lets everyone know how each person is feeling, and we can treat them accordingly.) Favorite color? Name? Age? Song? Favorite place? And so on...

In depth circle work branches into the theme or topic to be explored and discovered. For

Module One we will be focusing on Self Love questions and how it relates to us as a whole being. (More on this in modules 5, 6 and 7)

There are a total of eight classes and modules to complete the stacking modules: This is Module One Self Love. The following page has an example of a safe and brave space contract. In stacking Module Seven, you will set up your own **Safe and Brave Spaces Guidelines.**

To begin this workshop we invite you to our Safe and Brave Space guidelines as written by our founder Heidi Little, M. Ed. The safe and brave space guidelines set up the space for us to begin our exploration into Self Love Module One.

And so we begin. Please read **An Invitation To Safe and Brave Space:**

An Invitation To Safe And Brave Space

AS WE COME TOGETHER WE CREATE SAFE
AND BRAVE SPACE.
BECAUSE WE KNOW WE CREATE
'"SAFE AND BRAVE SPACE"
WE WILL CONSCIOUSLY CHOOSE TO BE A PART
OF, AND STAND UP FOR, SAFE AND BRAVE SPACE.

WE EXIST IN THE REAL WORLD.
WHERE THOUGHTS BECOME THINGS,
AND EVERY ACTION HAS A REACTION.
WE ALL CARRY SCARS, AND
WE HAVE ALL CAUSED WOUNDS,

HERE WE ARE IN BALANCE.

WE SEEK TO TURN DOWN THE VOLUME
OF THE OUTSIDE WORLD,
AND EXPLORE OUR INNER KNOWING,
OUR VOICES, OUR CHOICES, OUR KNOWLEDGE,
OUR UNIQUE GIFTS, MISSIONS AND PURPOSE.
AND WORK INDIVIDUALLY, AND TOGETHER.

WE CALL EACH OTHER TO MORE TRUTH AND LOVE.
WE HAVE THE RIGHT TO CHOOSE OUR DELIVERY.
WE HAVE THE RIGHT TO SHINE WITHIN OUR HEARTS
WITH THE LIGHT OF ONE THOUSAND GOLDEN SUNS.
HERE WE DO SUPPORT AND UPLIFT BOLD CHOICES,

HERE WE REALIZE EVERYONE IS IN THE ACT OF
CREATING AT ALL TIMES,

THE ART OF BECOMING.

An Invitation To Safe And Brave Space

CREATIVITY IS LOVE, I AM LOVE,
WE ARE LOVE.
AND TOGETHER WE WILL CREATE SOMETHING
BEAUTIFUL AND TANGIBLE

WE MAY DISAGREE, BUT WE WILL DO SO
WITH KINDNESS.

IT MAY NOT ALWAYS BE WHAT WE WISH IT TO BE,
AND THAT IS O.K.

BECAUSE WE ARE LEARNING TO WORK,
PLAY AND GROW TOGETHER.

SIDE BY SIDE, VOICE TO VOICE,
HEART TO HEART, LEARNING AND MASTERING

OUR THOUGHTS, FEELINGS, BELIEFS
AND DELIVERY TRANSFORM THINGS,

WE TAKE RESPONSIBILITY FOR THIS UNDERSTANDING

WE BELIEVE IN OURSELVES, IN RELATION TO
FAMILY, COMMUNITY AND OUR WORLD
WE ARE ARISING TO OUR HIGHEST HEART CALLING
AND INNER GUIDANCE SYSTEM
WE ARE
ACTIVE IN THE POWER OF THE PRESENT MOMENT.
WE DO OUR BEST, AND THAT IS WHAT COUNTS..

HEIDI LITTLE, M. ED
FOUNDER HEART BASED EDUCATION AND THE CENTER FOR
ADVANCEMENT IN HEART BASED EDUCATION 05.2025

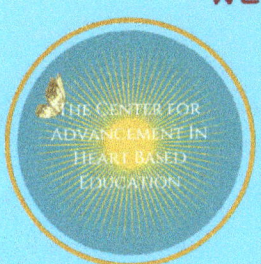

www.HeartBasedEd.org

Ensure, everyone agrees to the 'Safe and Brave Space" guidelines.

INTRODUCE YOURSELF: Whether you are completing this module Self Paced, or are a part of a group or cohort: Write out or speak out loud your introduction. How do you introduce yourself. Name, passion, and what brought you to the work? 1-3 minute shares.

Facilitated Classes: Here we will have a short introduction of each member of the training. Light facilitation is encouraged. Name, passion, and what brought you to the work? 1-3 minutes.

Heart Based Education Defined:

The Center for Advancement in Heart Based Education

Heart Based Education is a whole-person approach to learning, based in the heart, that nurtures and empowers every part of a person and their life—heart, body, mind, and spirit. Through activations/meditations, meaningful activities, and personal exploration, it helps individuals understand themselves more deeply, strengthen their relationships and purpose, in right relation to their family, community, and the world. It's about becoming one's full, authentic self—and supporting others to do the same.

www.HeartBasedED.org

SELF LOVE EXPLORATION

SELF LOVE DEFINITION FROM THE CENTER FOR ADVANCEMENT IN HEART BASED EDUCATION: Self love is a positive, uplifting, accepting, compassionate, kind, and supportive way of being with self. It is an intimate and deep connection with self.

This portion of the module can be done solo, in a group, online, or in person.

You will need a pen/pencil/art supplies/ paper/notebook. We write out this portion because it supports creating new neural pathways in the brain, and discovers old neural pathways.

Following are a series of questions. Please answer fully and give as much time as is required to do a deep dive. There is always a point where participants believe they are done. Push past this and allow another minute or five to the overall time spent on each question.

Solo Work: Ready yourself with this module, your preferred method of writing, and notebook.

Group: Begin by calling in a circle and remind participants of the purpose and the guidelines

- We do not speak out of turn
- Each person's time to share is theirs to share, and we respect others' time who are listening, as we are respected while we share
- No feedback
- We are all here showing up in the moment

Online Education: Set the tone for the space, set the boundaries of the safe and brave container. We begin by calling in a circle. As we all share clockwise - name, age, favorite color, and one word to describe how we are feeling today - we get into a safe space where everyone is heard. Lightly facilitate this circle experience.

SELF LOVE GUIDED QUESTIONS. TAKE AS LONG AS REQUIRED TO ANSWER. THE ENTIRE EXPERIENCE COULD TAKE UP TO 50 MINUTES.

1. What does self love feel like for you personally?
2. What do you feel self love looks like?
3. What does self love sound like?
4. Can you locate your inner voice of self love? What does he/she/pronoun sound like?
5. What does self love show up like?
6. What is Love In Action?
7. What does love in action look like?
8. What does love in action sound like?
9. What does love in action feel like?

Groups: Have an open conversation around each of these topics.

We will spend most of our time going through this portion of the embodiment training. Connecting the mind and the emotional body. A minimum of 40 minutes is spent in conversation on these topics and, as we talk and move through it, understanding and choices will be made by all in regards to how self love works and enhances their lives.

Facilitators may extend the exploration into present common societal factors or events, around self care, connection etc, and coming back to the heart and self love being the docking station, the platform, and the stage from which to spring forth into the life we are living and actively creating. Self love and a direct connection to the heart is the key to a happy and healthy life.

Take A 15 Minute Break Here:

Here we dive into the heart anchoring activation. Prepare yourself (Students) by asking them to get comfortable, and ready to proceed with the activation. No cell phones, no interruptions.

ACTIVITY #3 CORE MODULE ONE TEACHING/EMBODIMENT PRACTICE AND TOOL.

Seed of Light Activation/Meditation™

This can take up to 25 min to compete

We begin by breathing in the love, and breathing out the love.

Breathe in the love. Breathe out the love.

Breathe in the love. Breathe out the love.

Breathe in the love. Breathe out the love.

Bring your hands up to your heart, left hand over heart, right hand over heart

Imagine a seed of light in your heart

What does it look like? Is it deep and vast? multifaceted? Soft and glowing?

breathe in the love, and breathe out the love

As you breathe in the love, and breathe out the love that seed of light grows and glows

Breathe in the love. Breathe out the love

Breathe in the love. Breathe out the love

Breathe in the love. Breathe out the love

The light expands as you breathe

The seed of light fills your whole heart

Breathe in the love. Breathe out the love

The light lovingly expands to fill your chest

Breathe in the love. Breathe out the love

The seed of light grows and flows up into your shoulders

down your arms, and into your hands

Breathing in the love. Breathing out the love

The heart light grows to fill your throat, and up your neck into your face and head

Breathe in the love. Breathe out the love

The light is filling your upper body, flowing into your stomach and down through your

organs

Breathe in the love, breathe out the love

The seed of light in your heart grows and glows, and flows down

into your pelvis and your hips.

Breathe in the love. Breathe out the love.

The light flows lovingly down into your thighs and into your knees

Breathe in the love.Breathe out the love.

Lovingly flowing down into your calves and into your ankles

Breathing in the love. Breathing out the love.

The light flows down into your feet

All the way to your toes

Breathe in the love. Breathe out the love.

From the tippy toes to the top of your head.

Whole body heart light

Breathe in the love. Breathe out the love.

Imagine the seed of light in your heart, glowing. Feeling your heart connection.

We are going to spend a few minutes here.

Breathe in the love, breathe out the love.

Continue breathing in the love and out the love

(Rest here in safe and brave space for a few minutes, periodically reminding your

participants to breathe in the love and out the love)

imagining the seed of light beginning to grow and expand.

Breathe in the peace, breathe out the peace, breathe in the love, breathe out the love.

Stay connected to the seed of light in your heart. Focus on it.

Breathe in the love, breathe out the love.

Here we are going to look at expanding our light.

Breathe in the love, breathe out the love.

Bring your focus to the seed and the light in your heart.

Which feels better? To keep the light small and contained just to your body? Or to reach

out with it?

How far can you reach?

Breathe in the love, breathe out the love.

Breathe in the love. Breathe out the love.

Bringing our focus back to your heart space.

Breathe in the love, breathe out the love.

Continue to breathe here for some moments.

Focusing on the seed of light in your heart space.

Breathe in the love. Breathe out the love

Breathing in the love, breathing out the love.

(Here gently guide your participants to give themselves a welcome home massage. Go slowly.)

Keeping everything going, gently bring your hands together and rub them

Create some warmth and heart in your hands

We are going to gently bring our hands up to your face and

give yourself a little face message.

Forehead, temples, cheeks, above the lip, below the lip, and then to the ears where

nerves for your whole body reside.

Give yourself some time here.

Gently and lovingly massage your ears, and your earlobes.

Rub your arms,

Run your hands over your chest, back, bottom, legs, and feet.

Lastly, rub the hands together until you create warmth.

Create a small imaginary ball of white light between your palms, roll the ball in your

hands.

Gently pull your palms away from each other, essentially stretching the ball, coming

together with the palms and apart. Can you feel the stretchy substance? That is your

Chi! Our bodies' energy!

Gently bring your hands back up to your heart. Right hand and then left hand.

Breathe in the love. Breathe out the love.

Breathe in the love. Breathe out the love.

Breathe in the love. Breathe out the love.

Gently wiggle your toes. And wiggle your nose.

Gently open your eyes.

Note To Learners:

This is a life transforming exercise. Please be gentle with yourself and with others.
Please tell your children/adults/classes that this is a big deal -a cultivation - and that
they now have the tool/technique to bring in peace, love, balance, and harmony any
time they choose To restore self. To harmonize self. And to balance their bodies easily.
This is the platform, stage, or docking station for their human experience.

We complete the exercise with I AM statements.

We say to ourselves:

I am love.

I am beautiful.

I am safe.

I am loved.

Wiggle your nose and wiggle your toes.

Open your eyes when you are ready.

Remember!!! All one needs to do to get back to this space is breathe in the love and

breathe out the love.

GUIDED AUDIO VERSION OF THE SEED OF LIGHT MEDITATION/VISUALIZATION™

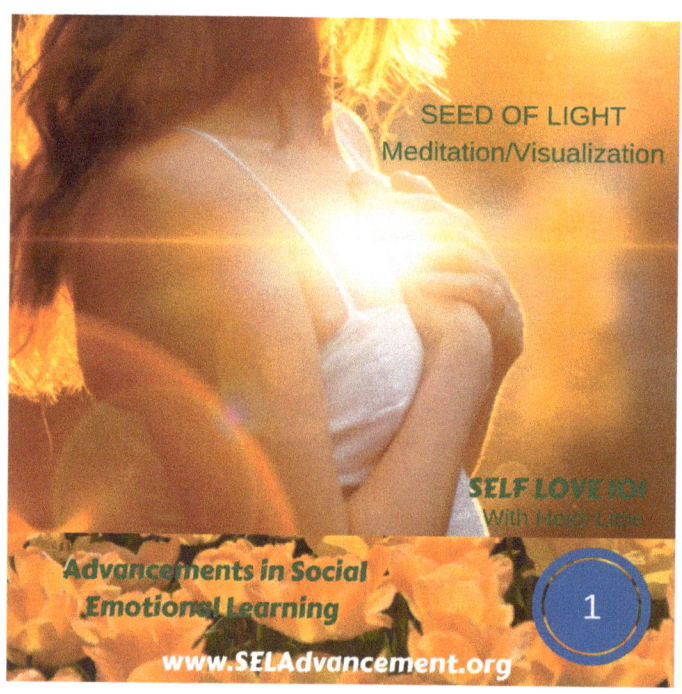

Available here:
https://seladvancement.bandcamp.com/album/self-love-1-seed-of-light-meditation-and-visualization

GROUPS: When all are ready, hold the space to have a lightly facilitated discussion about how this activity felt and what their experiences were. This is voluntary, not mandatory.

Give a space for participants to describe their experiences. Nothing is right or wrong.

Here you can explore and have a further conversation about how this tool/technique could potentially transform the person positively. Explore the effects on self, family, community and the world. Support self expression, coming home to self, the right to feel, and to acknowledge what is going on for each person.

Speak to and through this activation. We bring our higher power to ourselves and into our bodies. We facilitate a connection that is paramount to a happy healthy lifestyle. **The seed of light activation connects participants directly to their hearts.**

This is the baseline and most important teaching in this course. Everything builds on this technique. It is your first and "go to" tool.

A deep connection, and the acknowledgement and understanding that self love is important for every human being - that this can prevent and solve:problems, imbalances, and crises with self, in the family, in the community, in the classroom, and in the world. A deep connection to self cultivates an appropriate skill set to maintain a healthy and balanced lifestyle, in connecting to the heart, and as a support that, if cultivated, can prevent imbalances which affect mental health, suicide rates, drug use, depression, gun violence, poverty, hardship and any of life's challenges.

We use Self Love Practices to transform and release anxiety, depression, loneliness, anger and resentment. Self love practice builds resilience, uplifts and empowers, inspires, ignites, fuels creativity, interdependence, cooperation, promotes a sense of belonging,of connection, of safety; brings balance to body, mind, and spirit, and is the ultimate mindfulness practice - the foundational technique to restore and replenish.

Having the right to just be in alignment with self is the best gift you can give to yourself and to others. Teaching self love is the single most important thing we can learn, understand, and do to foster a healthy, happy, balanced person and life.

Thank your participants with depth and grace. Congratulations!

NOTE: The accompanying self-work will solidify the practice, embodiment, and pedagogy.

CERTIFICATION AT HOME REQUIREMENTS:

The SEED OF LIGHT™ exercise and its embodiment is KEY. To become certified, you must successfully embody these four parts:

1. Hold this activation for a minimum of fifteen minutes per day for the entire seven days, and continue the practice throughout the next seven certifications.(This is why we call them stacking certifications)

2. The second portion of this certification is to journal your experience. Write down how you feel, and what is shifting for you?

3. The third part is to create ten power statements per day, pertaining to your growth and the possibilities and new directions that come in for you.

4. One instructional video of you self guiding the Seed of Light Heart Connection activity.
5. Connect with your inner voice for self love, and explore that relationship.

To complete your certification send your written work and one instructional video of you guiding the seed of light activation, into a dropbox folder. Each facilitator may have a certain way to organize student assessments. Please upload all jpegs and videos at one time. Email the requirements for this certification to centerforadvancementsel@gmail.com **Make your header: Certification Assessments Module One (Your Name). Please have all materials in 24 hours before your next Module Training.**

Participants **will receive their certificate of completion for each module upon successful completion of the assessment components.**

The Center for Advancement in Heart Based Education™, congratulates you on this important work you are doing for self and the people you will support in restoration and self love.

There are further supplemental materials, trainings, workshops and curriculum available on www.HeartBasedED.org

Further Supports:

1. Module TWO Be The Medicine, The Medicine Wheel Exploration Technique™
2. 14 thematic, empowerment activity platforms for youth, parents, educators and humanity that can be used as a year long support for SEL curriculum www.internationalchildrensmonth.com
3. Want to make a difference? Join a team of professionals who are working on transforming society into a more equitable and just world? Or pad your resume? Try www.we.net
4. MODULE A MONTH www.HeartBasedED.org
5. MONTHLY MEMBERSHIP www.HeartBasedED.org
6. BECOME A TRAINER IN HEART BASED EDUCATION www.HeartBasedED.org

THE CENTER FOR ADVANCEMENT IN HEART BASED EDUCATION
OFFERS HEART BASED, IMPACT SPEAKING, 8 WEEK TRAINING WORKSHOPS,
CLASSES, MEMBERSHIPS, PARTNER CURRICULUM AND LICENSING, TRAINING AND
EXPERIENCES SINCE 1993

For Personal and Professional Development for all ages. Whether you are a parent, a CEO, an NGO, a humanitarian worker, a child/youth or teen, we have a turnkey heart based development set of tools, techniques, and inspirations for you. Our stacking modules are our framework:

1: Self-Love Module One/Certification One™
2: Be the Medicine Module Two/Certification Two™
3: Identity Module Three/Certification Three™
4: Self in Relation to Community Module Four/Certification Four™
5: Self in Relationship with the World and Universe Module Five/Certification Five™
6: The Classroom and Community as a Social System Module Six/Certification Six™
7: Creating Safe and Brave Spaces Module Seven/Certification Seven™
8: Chart and Launch Your Next Level Journey Module Eight/Certification Eight™

New Classes Begin ongoing https://www.heartbaseded.org

A note to registrants:

We know how challenging today's current landscape is. We have created a heart-centered approach over the past 25 years, that includes a curriculum, focused on the heart of each person, with over 30 years of implemented activities, and now the revitalization of soft skills, and empowerment techniques, that elevates and supports our students.

We stand in the present and look to the future with hope for the support, healing, and restoration of healthy, happy people, and for inclusive caring, supportive communities, and societies. We have developed a turnkey, 25 year vetted set of social-emotional learning modules/manuals full of a variety of techniques, and tools, using eight stacking, turnkey instructional modules. to support you and your staff/clients/students on an exploration of self, in relation to family, community and the world.

We feel best when we know who we are, and our purpose and internal connections are intact. What are your goals, gifts, mission and purpose? With over 30 years on the ground in three countries and all types of classrooms, and cultures, we feel our progressive, heart based education design and implementation experience has and is answering the needs of our past, current and future generations. Through a literal connection to the heart, and an exploration of the self, in relation to family, community, and the world, we are happy to share our modules and workshops/certifications.

Here are three ways you can get involved, certified, or learn more!

OUR SPECIALTY: ONLINE TRAINING TRAIN THE TRAINER REGISTER TODAY
www.HeartBasedED.org

WE CAN COME TO YOU. BOOK A WORKSHOP, IMPACT SPEAKING ENGAGEMENT AND/OR TRAINING SESSION TODAY!
centerforadvancementsel@gmail.com

Our module/workshops are a blend of practical hearts-based practices, independent written/creative activities, group discussions, and cultivating creative and inspiring work that centers around the exploration of self. Including the heart, as well as our body, mind and spirit, intellect, and communication skills, grounded by exploration in goals, talents, gifts, and what inspires us most. We have been teaching these practices, tools and techniques internationally with all types of cultural backgrounds, in all types of educational settings, and we have now created even more to support the people in our lives, working with children, youth, and adults of all ages: 45 Minute to 3 hour experiences/classes and workshops.

Modules can be done in a 8 week cohort, self paced through our membership platform or as an intensive 1-2 day experience.

Module 1: Self-Love: Self love is something that we cultivate within ourselves and as educators in others. The landscape of education is transforming along with us. We realize the importance of Social Emotional Learning. Through understanding self, family, community and the world, focused on our own personal self love, we begin to create a different landscape that works for us individually and because of that, works for others. Based on the basic principles, guidelines, and ethics of Social Emotional Learning, this module/certification explores tools and techniques that have been crafted over 30 years of Social Emotional Learning experiences that inspire and enhance a deep connection to self. Let us be happy in our bodies, as we cultivate resilience, inner peace, breath work, mindfulness, feeling like we belong, with empathy, compassion, and a skill set to navigate challenging times with grace and ease, while loving ourselves and each other. Complete with assessments of written and video components. We lead with the heart. These embodiment practices, tools and techniques are the foundation, the deep healing, and the restoration to our stacking curriculum. Experience literal heart-based connection, breath, while cultivating inspiration and an activated power of presence.

Self Love Workshop One: Explores techniques and tools utilized and taught over 30 years in three countries, and internationally! Students have found a deep connection with self, how to maintain and cultivate that connection at any time, as we explore our deep and rich inner world, and fill up our lives. Group discussions, and some real world applications that allow the student a safe and brave space to fully explore and come home to self, and leave with activation techniques that can be used as daily practice, or as a deep reset as we navigate life with joy, self control, and love. This class includes the Seed of Light Activation.

Module 2: Mapping Out Self: Connection to our inner guidance system is something that we cultivate within ourselves and, as educators, in others. The landscape of education is transforming along with us. We realize the importance of Heart Based Education. Through understanding self, family, community, and the world, focused on our own personal exploration and discovery, we begin to create a different landscape that works for us individually and because of that, works for others. This module/certification is a guide to and through embodiment practices, tools, and techniques that have been tested and proven effective over the past 30 years in education settings internationally, for all ages and beliefs. We have spent many years training bodies and minds. It is time to focus on the inner guidance system, and our deep connection with self. Through mapping, things become clear. When we actively participate in our healing, through written and creative work, we can literally see what we are thinking, feeling and addressing with self. The Center for Advancement has a unique and age-old tool of utilizing the medicine wheel to understand, explore and determine what is important to us. As we design and commit to our lives and what we are cultivating, natural healing occurs. The companion manual for this module is Be The Medicine, The Medicine Wheel Exploration Technique. Utilizing a technique based in mapping, participants will be guided into exploration and cultivation of personal dreams, hopes, and goals, while exploring areas that are necessary for our health and wellness, wholeness, and success. We will explore and come to understand self, family, community, and the world, while witnessing and experiencing what it feels like to 'hold safe and brave space' for self and others.

Be The Medicine: Workshop Two: Utilizes the small group environment, the medicine wheel exploration technique, and rich, exploratory mapping to actively create, and put down on paper however the student wishes, their deepest inspirations, dreams, desires, present reality, and future realities. To understand self, and facilitate the highest outcome for their lives. Complete with another infamous activation to bring self home to the heart. Explore with the medicine wheel exploration technique, designed to set you free, and continue to support your life, love and happiness as you transform and grow. This class includes the Seed of Light Activation and the Life Force Activation.

Module 3: Identity: Who are you in actuality? How did you form your opinion of yourself? What areas do you wish to cultivate or transform? This module is about discovering the greatest you, and what fuels and inspires you. The module uses guided exploration through independent and group questions, as we explore: What is yours to do and to be? Our identities can be confusing at times. As families, societies, and the media tell us who we are or who we should be, the real work and creativity here is in self exploration into how we as individuals really work and who we really want to cultivate as self showing up in the world. Here we explore choices and options, and make some solid decisions based on what brings us joy, uncovering and solidifying our gifts, supporting our happiness, and a sense of well being. We begin to explore the things we have in common with others, and how to fit in naturally with appreciation for ourselves, fitting in within a complex social system.

IDENTITY: Workshop Three: Is a kindness workshop, a compassion workshop and a self love workshop all in one. Exploring through the medicine wheel, group conversations, and reciprocity as water beings on a water planet, we will seek out and identify the motivating forces in our identity from our upbringing, society and self talk, and reinvent, conceptualize and activate, a present version of who and what we are on the planet at this time. When we know self, love self, and make decisions based in our highest outcome, we create new timelines, new worlds, and a new future, that is in alignment with our gifts, inspirations and desires. You decide who you are. This class includes The Oneness Activation.

Module 4: Self in Relation to Community: When we have deeply explored and rooted our self love, our inner guidance system and our understanding of our personal identity, we have set a foundation that is empowered and centered, balanced and whole to move out into the world. We have embodied techniques of resilience. Through social emotional learning we realize the importance of what we cultivate within ourselves and, as educators/community members, in others. How do we fit in with our community? How do we fit in with Society? What are the points that work to support us being "a part of" and "included in?" How is it that we come to feel included, and like we are contributing? What would we like to bring forward more readily and embody more often in these areas? Participants will seek to understand, cultivate, and embody their best sense of self in relation to community. Explore what it is to feel a part of, to feel connected with others, and work within a healthy and balanced body, mind and spirit.

Self In Relation To Community: Workshop Four: We came here to be together, let's be courageous and brave in our enrichment, and our community. This workshop explores "Tending our personal field." Here you will learn how to clear your energy field from the unconscious connections that happen throughout our day and lives. If you have a job that requires you to be around people, this one is essential for you. Learn how to fill up your personal cup, and keep it clear so the days of drain are over. We will also explore the safe and brave spaces concept, as well as restorative circle work.

Module 5: Self in Relationship with the World and Universe: Being a part of something greater than ourselves. Is it love, compassion, and kindness, or perhaps higher power, spirit, or creator? How about your ancestral relations? Grandmothers and Grandfathers, whether physically present here or not -- we are all connected. What is the concept of WE or oneness? How can this activity of exploration and embodying these concepts support us on our journey? Creativity, inspiration, understanding where we come from, in order to move forward. This module is more expansive and spiritually based. It is based in self love, non violent communication, and an understanding of self in relation to the universe we are a part of.

Self In Relation To The World And Universe: How do we begin to craft and prepare to take our gifts, messages and creations out to the world? We will explore, and make some choices in this module. The meditation and guided visualization in this module connects the learner through self to the planet and the universe. Continuing the support of working with breath and imagery to create a relationship with our natural world, space, and the spirit of oneness.

Module 6: The Classroom and the World as a Social System: How do we work Heart Based Education and Heart Based Exploration into a classroom or community setting? Everywhere can be a classroom. What is the social setting? How can it progress? How are you setting up your classroom or education space? How will you utilize the tools you have learned in the previous modules and share them in your community, through your work? How do different personality types and people/personality types play off each other? We will explore the classroom within the larger framework of schools, education systems, society and communities. How to naturally navigate a classroom filled with personalities, with gifts, and a sense of identity. How can we empower the people in our groups, networks, classrooms, and organizations to show up as their best selves, and take part, to create a good team. Remembering that a good team is made up of very unique people, all with different skills and abilities. Participants will learn embodiment practices, tools, and techniques to foster a solid foundation of self in relation to the classroom, and how we foster that space for others. As well as being introduced to "Restorative Circle Practice". This is transformative to our gun violence narrative we are experiencing today. People will make very different choices if they have the opportunity to find out who they are, and how to cultivate their best selves, and if given time to understand others in their classrooms, communities, and settings. Giving the space that is desperately being called out for to be heard, seen, and understood. Through restorative circle work, we can transform fear, and loneliness into inspired creativity, and a sense of belonging. (This is also our Emergency Action Plan. We would be happy to forward the complete module to you at your request.)

The Classroom and Community/World as a Social System: We require leaders in this time to hold safe and brave space, and have the ability to release, receive and restore. This certification centers around your personal gifts, and inner callings and how to continue to explore, shape and create them so they can be shared with others, you can be of service to whomever you decide to support.

Module 7: Creating Safe and Brave Spaces: Safe and brave spaces are designed and cultivated. How can we create those spaces to foster the learning outcomes of Heart Based Education that we have been cultivating within ourselves, in our students, and in our communities? What type of classroom do you want to foster? What type of community do you want to foster? What are the boundaries in your personal framework that support you and which keep you and your students and clients flourishing, and being safe, and brave? Cultivating your safe and brave space guidelines are the main focus of this module/certification. Participants will determine what that looks like, feels like, and sounds like, as well as drafting their safe and brave space guidelines to be implemented. Also learn how to craft, and recreate/teach, and design these guidelines for your offerings, community and global spaces.

Module 8: Chart and Launch Your Next Level Journey: This module/certification is all about you. What have you learned? Come to terms with? How would you like to continue to foster your development moving forward? What class, book, workshop, speaking engagement calls to you? How will you implement all of this into your work? Participants will determine goals and design the implementation to successfully accomplish those goals. This is creating your Heart Based Action plan, or your education plan, life plan, or dream plan. Whether it is your own program, or moving forward in community, or with your family or classroom, or perhaps to become a certified instructor/educator with The Center for Advancement in Heart Based Education. We lead with the heart.

All workshops come with a PDF of the modules, and a certificate of completion. A Diploma in Heart Based Education may be granted after all work has been turned in, and each module certificate has been completed. An overall completion of all 8 modules is granted to those who arrive on time, do their work to the best of their ability, and show the true spirit of Heart Based Education, and dedication to the work.

Upon completion of all eight modules participants will:

- Have a direct connection to your heart, and inner guidance system
- Know your gifts, mission and purpose
- Know tools and techniques that can be used as daily practice and have the ability to teach those techniques to others.
- Embody breath work and activities that will connect humans to their hearts and foster a deeper connection to self.
- Have cultivated and understand compassion, empathy and group communication.
- Know tools and techniques to tap into the inner guidance system and share these techniques.
- Have the tools to maintain a healthy and happy energetically enhanced life.
- Unlock and tap into their creativity.
- Focus, attention, intention
- Fully explore, gifts, and abilities, and which ones of these gifts and abilities they are most in alignment with.
- Understand themselves in relation to family, community and the world.
- Have the tools to be happy, healthy, and balanced people.
- Have cultivated and explored: self-awareness, self-management, social awareness, relationship skills, and responsible decision-making.
- Be awarded certificates in successfully completed modules.

- Have the potential to be accredited and supported to begin or expand their Social Emotional Learning teaching journey, with practicum and mentorship opportunities, locally and internationally.
- Earn the opportunity to move forward and become a certifying trainer for the Center for Advancement in Heart Based Education
- Become a member of the Heart Based Education community
- Potential to be granted listing on our website as a Center for Advancement in Heart Based Education as a Certified Educator.
- Most importantly, each participant will have a new set of tools and techniques to utilize during lifes day to day challenges, and be prepared for resilience and a well balanced lifestyle for the future

Mission: We are International Humanity, from all walks of life, implementing Heart Based Education, while raising the bar of/for love, care and respect, for ourselves, and all our relations. www.HeartBasedEd.org

Schedule a 30 min meeting to discuss opportunities:

https://calendly.com/seladvancements/new-meeting

Get in touch now: Heidi Little, M. Ed 512-799-9807

Email: book@heidilittle.com

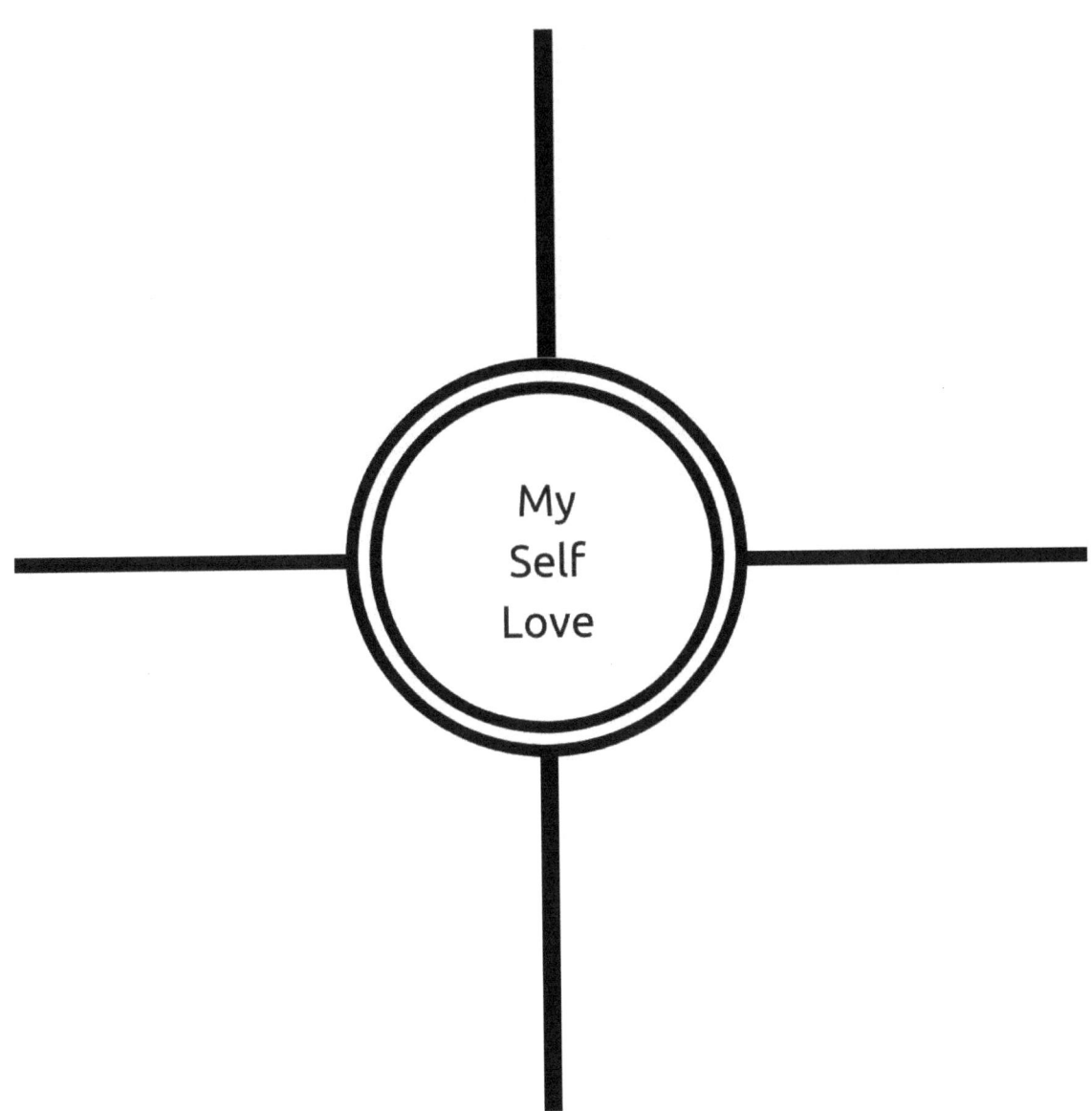

Work with this medicine wheel by adding what you feel best supports the center with 4 major areas of importance to cultivation and support of your self love. Using the four points beginning in the east, and moving in a clockwise circle to the south, west, and north, map out the most important things at this moment regarding cultivating your self love.

NOTES

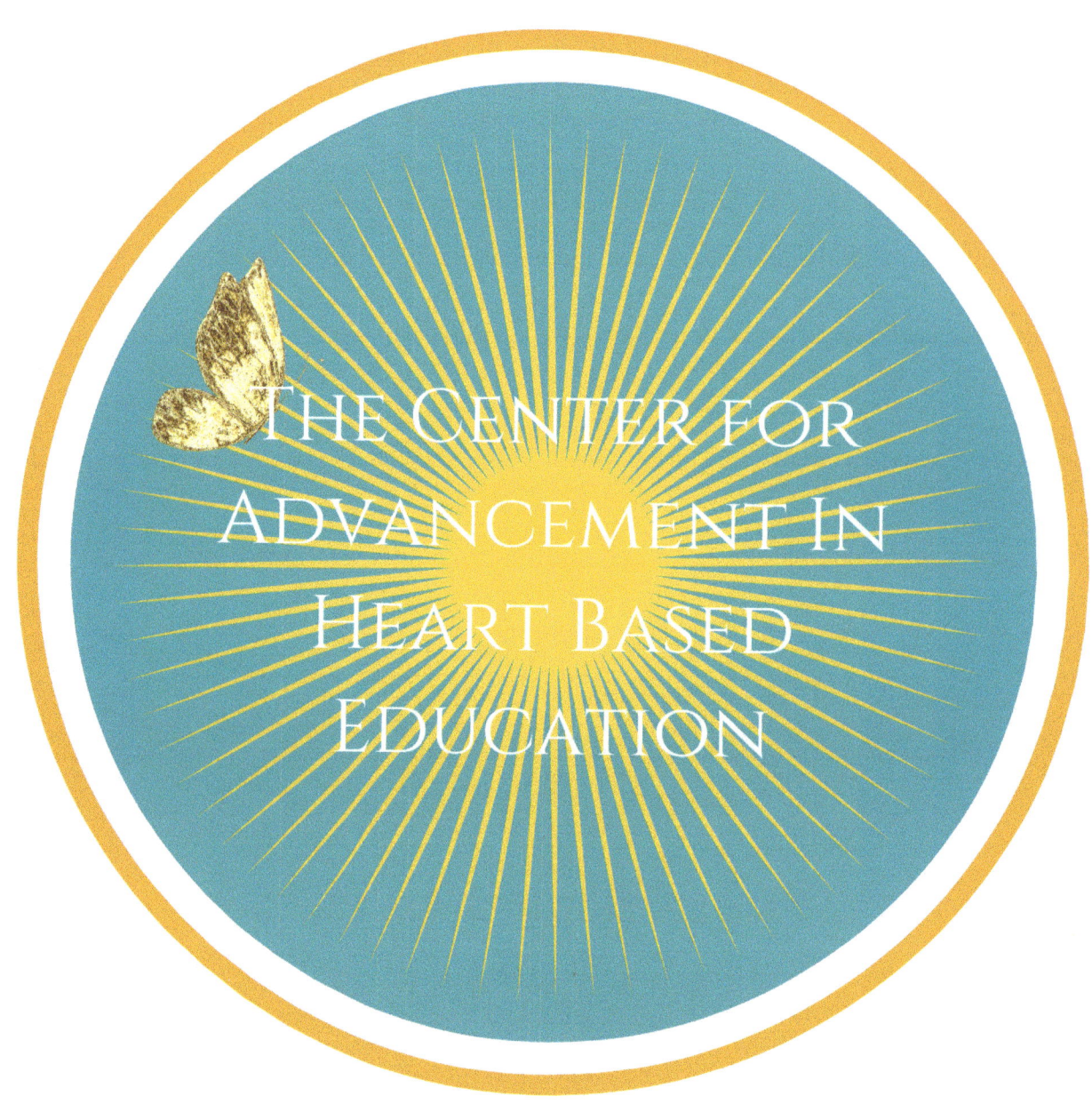